PROSTATITIS NUTRITION FOR NEWLY DIAGNOSED

Optimize Your Diet To Combat Prostatitis -
Understand The Key Nutrients, Foods To Avoid,
And Lifestyle Changes For Lasting Wellness

DR. ERIC TRISTAN

CONTENTS

DISCLAIMER

The information provided in this book, is intended for informational purposes only. The content is not intended to be a substitute for professional medical advice, diagnosis, or treatment. Always seek the advice of your physician or other qualified health provider with any questions you may have regarding a medical condition. Never disregard professional medical advice or delay in seeking it because of something you have read in this book.

The author of this book has made reasonable efforts to ensure that the information provided is accurate and up-to-date at the time of publication. However, the author makes no representations or warranties of any kind, express or implied, about the completeness, accuracy, reliability, suitability, or availability of the information contained within these pages.

Any reliance you place on the information provided in this book is strictly at your own risk. The author shall not be liable for any loss, injury, or damage arising from the use of this book or the information contained herein.

The mention or reference to any individuals, products, websites, organizations, or other names within this book does not imply endorsement by the author. The inclusion of such references is solely for informational purposes and does not constitute an endorsement or recommendation.

Furthermore, the author disclaims any association or affiliation with any individuals, products, websites, organizations, or other names mentioned in this book.

It is important to consult with a qualified healthcare professional before making any dietary or lifestyle changes, especially if you have a medical condition. Each individual's health situation is unique, and what works for one person may not work for another.

Again, the information provided in this book is not intended to diagnose, treat, cure, or prevent any disease or health condition. Always seek the advice of a physician or other qualified health provider regarding any medical questions or concerns you may have.

Thank you for your understanding and for taking the necessary precautions when considering the information presented in this book.

ABOUT THIS BOOK

"Prostatitis Nutrition" serves as an all-encompassing manual that sheds light on the pivotal significance of nutrition in the treatment and control of prostatitis, a medical condition that disproportionately impacts the male population. This book begins with a perceptive preface that establishes the context for a comprehensive examination of prostatitis and its multifaceted nature. The 'Understanding Prostatitis' section offers readers a comprehensive understanding of the condition, laying a strong groundwork for the subsequent discussions. A central theme emphasized in this book is the 'Importance of Nutrition in Prostatitis Management,' which clarifies the substantial influence that dietary decisions have on symptom relief and the promotion of prostate health as a whole.

The following chapters provide practical advice, beginning with "Dietary Guidelines for Prostatitis," which delineates precise dietary suggestions that are crucial for the management of the condition. This book 'Foods to Avoid for Prostatitis' and 'Anti-Inflammatory Foods for Prostatitis' provide readers with additional information that enables them to make well-informed dietary choices. This book further delves into the topic of 'Nutritional Supplements for Prostatitis,' providing insights into supplementary products that could potentially enhance dietary approaches.

In 'Hydration and its Role in Prostatitis,' this book delves into the significance of sufficient fluid consumption, acknowledging the criticality of hydration. "Lifestyle Changes for Prostatitis Management" expands the discourse beyond dietary modifications to include comprehensive strategies for improving overall health. The relationship between prostate cancer and weight management is elucidated in "Prostatitis and Weight Management."

The emphasis is placed on practicality through the provision of 'Sample Meal Plans' and 'Recipes for Prostatitis-friendly Meals,' which furnish readers with tangible and executable instructions. This book

'Herbal and Natural Remedies' delves into alternative methodologies for the management of prostatitis, whereas the article 'Professional Guidance and Consultation' emphasizes the criticality of consulting authorities for informed counsel. In the final section of the book, "FAQs on Prostatitis Nutrition," frequent questions are answered and clarification is provided.

Fundamentally, "Prostatitis Nutrition" serves as an indispensable resource by elucidating the complex correlation that exists between nutrition and the management of prostatitis. This book's methodical structure, which is firmly rooted in data supported by scientific evidence, makes it an essential read for anyone grappling with the intricacies of prostatitis. It provides a clear path to better health and an elevated standard of living.

CHAPTER ONE

Introduction

Prostatitis, a medical condition distinguished by inflammation of the prostate organ, has the potential to induce a variety of distressing symptoms in men of every age. Although medical intervention is of utmost importance in the management of prostatitis, nutrition is equally significant in promoting prostate health as a whole and mitigating symptoms. This article delves into the significance of nutrition in the management of prostatitis, offering perspectives on dietary recommendations and lifestyle decisions that may promote prostate health.

Comprehension Of Prostatitis

Prostatitis is a prevalent yet intricate medical condition characterized by the inflammation of the prostate gland, which is a walnut-shaped, subabdominal organ in males. Each type of inflammation—acute, chronic, infectious, or non-infectious—presents a unique set of difficulties.

Acute bacterial prostatitis, which frequently arises from bacterial infections, is characterized by the abrupt onset of severe symptoms including fever, shivers, and severe pelvic pain.

Recurrent infections define chronic bacterial prostatitis, whereas chronic prostatitis/chronic pelvic pain syndrome (CP/CPPS) is the most prevalent manifestation that does not have a definitive bacterial etiology. Although asymptomatic inflammatory prostatitis may not manifest any discernible symptoms, it can be diagnosed by observing the presence of inflammation during diagnostic procedures.

Prostatitis is characterized by urinary tract pain or irritation in the pelvic region, urinary frequency or incontinence, and sexual dysfunction. A comprehensive strategy for managing prostatitis is imperative due to its multifaceted nature; in this regard, nutrition assumes a critical function in bolstering the overall health of the prostate.

Significance Of Nutrition In The Management Of Prostatitis

The management of prostatitis frequently necessitates an integration of medical interventions, modifications to one's lifestyle, and dietary adjustments. Nutrition, specifically, assumes a critical function in bolstering the immune system, mitigating inflammation, and advancing holistic health.

1. Prostatitis is frequently correlated with inflammation; therefore, implementing an anti-inflammatory diet may prove beneficial in symptom management. Typical omega-3 fatty acid-rich foods on this diet consist of hazelnuts, fatty fish (salmon, mackerel), and flaxseeds. It has been demonstrated that these nutrients possess anti-inflammatory properties, which may be advantageous for reducing prostate inflammation.

2. Antioxidant-Rich Foods: Antioxidants inhibit free radical-induced cell injury; therefore, prostate health needs to consume antioxidant-rich foods. Green tea,

berries, tomatoes, and broccoli are all rich in antioxidants. In addition to benefiting overall health, these foods also contribute to a diet that is prostate-friendly.

3. Protein Sources: Individuals diagnosed with prostatitis must prioritize the consumption of lean protein sources. By substituting lean meats, poultry, fish, tofu, and legumes for saturated fat, one can obtain essential amino acids. As excessive consumption of red and processed meats has been associated with an elevated risk of prostate problems, it may be advantageous to decrease one's ingestion of these foods.

4. Maintaining adequate hydration is critical for the health of the prostate. A sufficient water intake aids in the elimination of contaminants and preserves urinary function as a whole. It is recommended to restrict the intake of caffeinated and alcoholic beverages, as they have the potential to cause irritation to the prostate and worsen symptoms.

5. Precautions Regarding Trigger Foods: Specific foods have the potential to induce symptoms of prostatitis in certain individuals. Caffeine, acidic foods such as tomatoes, spicy foods, and alcohol may exacerbate symptoms in some patients. Identification and avoidance of these trigger foods are crucial for the management and prevention of symptom flare-ups.

Guidelines Regarding Dietary Prostatitis

Embracing a prostate-friendly diet necessitates purposeful decision-making that promotes holistic well-being and mitigates symptoms associated with prostatitis. Beneficial dietary recommendations for individuals managing prostatitis include the following:

1. Placing Emphasis on Plant-Based Foods: An eating regimen abundant in fruits, vegetables, whole cereals, and legumes supplies one with fiber, vital vitamins, and minerals. These dietary items derived from plants potentially possess anti-inflammatory

and antioxidant attributes that are advantageous for the health of the prostate.

2. Fatty fish, flaxseeds, chia seeds, and hazelnuts are all outstanding sources of omega-3 fatty acids that should be incorporated into one's diet. These nutrients have been linked to a decrease in inflammation and potentially aid in the management of prostatitis symptoms.

3. Maintain a Moderate Protein Intake: Fish, poultry, tofu, and legumes are examples of lean protein sources that should be prioritized over red and processed meats. Sufficient protein consumption is critical for optimal physiological functioning, and opting for lean alternatives can aid in symptom management while preventing the exacerbation of inflammation.

4. Maintaining proper hydration is essential for the health of the prostate. To mitigate the risk of prostate irritation, maintain a regular water intake throughout

the day and restrict the consumption of caffeinated and alcoholic beverages.

5. Restrict Trigger Food Intake: Recognize and abstain from consuming foods that have the potential to induce symptoms of prostatitis. Triggers such as spicy foods, caffeine, alcohol, and acidic foods are frequently encountered and can be mitigated to aid in the management of symptoms.

6. Consider Herbal Supplements: The potential benefits of certain herbal supplements, including saw palmetto and quercetin, in the management of prostatitis symptoms have been investigated. Before adding any dietary supplements to one's regimen, it is prudent to seek the guidance of a healthcare professional to verify that they are compatible with the individual's condition and treatment strategy.

7. It is advisable to maintain a healthy weight, as obesity has been associated with an elevated likelihood of developing prostate issues.

Weight maintenance through the adoption of a well-balanced diet and consistent participation in physical activity can effectively mitigate the likelihood of complications associated with prostatitis.

In summary, the management of prostatitis necessitates a comprehensive strategy, with nutrition serving as an essential component in promoting general prostate well-being.

Patients with prostatitis may experience symptom relief and an enhanced quality of life through the implementation of conscientious food selections, adherence to an anti-inflammatory and prostate-friendly diet, and adequate hydration.

It is recommended to seek personalized advice and guidance from healthcare professionals regarding dietary modifications, as with any medical condition.

CHAPTER TWO

Foods That Reduce Inflammation In Prostatitis

Prostatitis, an inflammatory condition affecting the prostate organ, can induce nausea and disrupt routine activities. Although medical interventions remain pivotal, supplementing with anti-inflammatory foods into one's diet may aid in symptom management and promote general prostate well-being.

1. Fatty fish, such as mackerel and salmon, contain omega-3 fatty acids which are known to exhibit significant anti-inflammatory properties. These lipids have the potential to mitigate prostatitis symptoms by reducing inflammation in the prostate.

2. Antioxidants, which are abundant in berries including blueberries and strawberries, protect against oxidative stress. Antioxidants aid in the neutralization of free radicals, thereby promoting prostate health and reducing inflammation.

3. Curcumin, the bioactive constituent of turmeric, possesses potent anti-inflammatory properties. It may be possible that supplementing with turmeric or incorporating it into curries could aid in the management of inflammation related to prostatitis.

4. Cruciferous vegetables, such as Brussels sprouts, broccoli, and cauliflower, contain compounds that aid in the body's natural detoxification. These vegetables potentially have anti-inflammatory and prostate health benefits.

5. Antioxidant lycopene, which is abundant in tomatoes, has been associated with prostate health. Lycopene may aid in the management of prostatitis symptoms by decreasing inflammation and oxidative stress, according to studies.

6. Green Tea: Green tea contains epigallocatechin gallate (EGCG), which is known to have anti-inflammatory properties. Consistent intake of green tea has the potential to mitigate inflammation and promote optimal prostate health.

7. Nuts and Seeds: Almonds, walnuts, and flaxseeds are rich in nutrients including omega-3 fatty acids. In addition to reducing inflammation, these foods may also supply vital nutrients for prostate health.

8. Olive Oil: Antioxidants and monounsaturated lipids, which are present in extra virgin olive oil, may have anti-inflammatory properties. Incorporating olive oil into salads or utilizing it as a primary culinary oil can prove to be advantageous when incorporated into an anti-inflammatory diet.

9. Ginger: For centuries, ginger has been utilized for its anti-inflammatory properties. Including ginger in one's dietary regimen, whether in the form of cooked ginger or ginger tea, has the potential to alleviate symptoms associated with prostatitis.

10. Probiotics are present in fermented foods such as sauerkraut, yogurt, and kefir, and they promote digestive health. A link between inflammation and gastrointestinal health is suggested by emerging

research; therefore, incorporating probiotics into your diet may indirectly benefit prostate health.

Avoidable Foods For Prostatitis

It is critical, when utilizing nutrition to treat prostatitis, to be cognizant of substances that could exacerbate inflammation or aggravate symptoms. Although individual reactions may differ, the following are overarching principles regarding food items to restrict or evade:

1. Spicy Foods Spicy foods, particularly those that contain chile peppers, may exacerbate the symptoms of prostatitis and irritate the prostate. Prohibiting the consumption of piquant foods may provide advantages for those who are afflicted with inflammation.

2. Caffeine has the potential to function as a diuretic, which may cause irritation to the bladder and worsen urinary symptoms that are commonly associated with prostatitis.

Coffee and tea are examples of caffeinated beverages that should be consumed in moderation.

3. Alcohol: Additionally, alcohol may cause urinary tract irritation and dehydration. Alcohol restriction can aid in hydration and decrease the likelihood that prostatitis symptoms will worsen.

4. Frequently, processed foods include excessive quantities of additives, sodium, and preservatives. Because these substances may contribute to inflammation, it is generally advised to consume whole, unprocessed foods.

5. A high consumption of red and processed meats has been linked to an elevated risk of inflammation. It may be preferable to consume lean protein sources such as poultry, salmon, or plant-based alternatives.

6. Some individuals with prostatitis may experience exacerbation of symptoms when consuming dairy products, especially full-fat varieties. Considering the possibility of experimenting with alternative milk

sources such as almond or soy milk could be beneficial.

7. There is evidence linking diets that are heavy in refined carbohydrates to inflammation. Reducing the intake of sweetened beverages, desserts, and munchies may aid in the management of prostatitis symptoms.

8. Certain individuals may develop hypersensitivity reactions to artificial compounds, such as preservatives and food colorings. It is beneficial to read food labels and select products with minimal additive content.

9. It is recommended that individuals who are susceptible to calcium oxalate kidney stones limit their consumption of high oxalate foods, such as beets, chocolate, and almonds, as they may contribute to urinary complications.

10. Saturated and trans fats, which are prevalent in processed and fried foods, have the potential to

contribute to inflammation when consumed in excessive quantities.

It is preferable to consume healthful lipids, such as those found in avocados and olive oil.

Supplemental Dietary Factors For Prostatitis

Specific nutritional supplements may be utilized in conjunction with a well-balanced diet to aid in the management of prostatitis symptoms. Before integrating supplements into your regimen, it is imperative to seek guidance from a healthcare professional, given that individual requirements may differ.

1. The potential anti-inflammatory properties of fish oil supplements containing omega-3 fatty acids have been suggested. Supplements of this nature may present a practical approach to augmenting one's omega-3 consumption, particularly in situations where dietary sources are restricted.

2. Quercetin, an anti-inflammatory flavonoid that is present in fruits and vegetables, possesses anti-inflammatory properties. Some research indicates that supplementation with quercetin may mitigate the symptoms of prostatitis.

3. Saw palmetto is a frequently utilized botanical supplement that is intended to promote prostate health. Although research is inconclusive, some men with prostatitis who take saw palmetto report symptomatic relief.

4. Sufficient quantities of vitamin D are critical for optimal bodily functioning, including that of the prostate. Your healthcare provider may recommend vitamin D supplements to bring your levels back within the healthy range if they are low.

5. Zinc: An essential mineral for prostate health. Although an overabundance of zinc can have detrimental effects on prostate health, ensuring sufficient levels through dietary means or supplementation may be beneficial.

6. Bromelain, an enzyme discovered in pineapple, possesses anti-inflammatory characteristics. Bromelain supplements have been reported to provide alleviation from prostatitis symptoms in some individuals.

7. Bromelain and Quercetin Combination: For a synergistic effect, certain supplements combine quercetin and bromelain. These mixtures may provide holistic assistance in the management of inflammation and symptoms associated with prostatitis.

8. Probiotic supplements have the potential to promote intestinal health, and recent studies indicate a potential correlation between digestive health and inflammation. Prostate health may be indirectly benefited by digestive health maintenance.

9. Green tea extract and other supplements abundant in polyphenols may offer anti-inflammatory and antioxidant properties. These supplements may

provide a practical means of augmenting one's consumption of polyphenols.

10. Cernilton, an extract sourced from rye grass pollen, is a dietary supplement that is occasionally employed to alleviate the symptoms associated with prostatitis. Before attempting this supplement, it is vital to consult a healthcare professional due to the ongoing research into its efficacy.

CHAPTER THREE

The Importance Of Hydration In Prostatitis

Constant hydration is essential for maintaining overall health and symptom management of prostatitis. Sustaining adequate hydration can yield numerous advantages for men afflicted with prostate inflammation:

1. Urinary health is influenced by adequate hydration, which reduces the concentration of substances that may irritate the prostate and bladder and helps maintain urinary flow. This is particularly crucial in the management of urinary symptoms that are linked to prostatitis.

2. Sufficient consumption of water facilitates the body's inherent detoxification mechanisms. By aiding in the elimination of debris and pollutants, hydration may reduce inflammation in the prostate.

3. Preventing Kidney Stone Formation: Dehydration has the potential to worsen symptoms of prostatitis

by contributing to the development of kidney stones. Maintaining adequate fluid consumption aids in the prevention of kidney stone formation.

4. Adequate hydration has the potential to augment the efficacy of medications that are prescribed for the treatment of prostatitis. By ensuring proper dilution and absorption, it maximizes the therapeutic effects of medications on inflammation and symptoms.

5. Mitigating Constipation: Prolonged constipation has the potential to exacerbate symptoms of prostatitis and impair pelvic floor function. Maintaining regular bowel movements through adequate water consumption reduces the risk of constipation.

6. For optimal cellular function, cells in the prostate and the rest of the body must be adequately hydrated. Cellular processes that are supported by hydration may contribute to the overall health of the prostate.

7. Enhanced General Well-Being: Dehydration can induce feelings of lethargy and an overall sense of malaise. Sufficient hydration enhances general health and may potentially augment the capacity to manage symptoms associated with prostatitis.

8. Electrolyte Balance: Hydration is an essential factor in preserving electrolyte balance, which is vital for the proper functioning of nerves and muscles. Electrolyte imbalances have the potential to generate distress and worsen symptoms that are commonly linked to prostatitis.

9. Mitigated Bladder Irritation: Hypohydration can lead to the production of concentrated urine, a substance that can exacerbate urinary symptoms and cause irritation to the bladder. Adequate hydration results in urine that is more diluted, which alleviates irritation.

10. Tailored Hydration Objectives: The optimal quantity of water consumed differs significantly between individuals. Age, weight, climate, level of

physical activity, and other variables all impact hydration requirements. It is critical to take into consideration the needs of your body and modify your fluid consumption accordingly.

As a result of the importance of nutrition in the management of prostatitis symptoms, an anti-inflammatory diet can positively impact prostate health as a whole. Assigning targeted supplements, avoiding potential irritants, and consuming nutrient-dense foods are all beneficial elements of a comprehensive approach that should be considered under the supervision of a healthcare professional. Furthermore, it is critical to ensure adequate hydration to promote urinary and overall health.

Constantly, personal reactions to dietary modifications and supplements may differ; therefore, it is imperative to seek guidance from a healthcare professional to customize recommendations to particular circumstances and requirements.

Prostatitis Nutrition For Promoting Prostate Health

The effect of prostatitis, an inflammation of the prostate organ, on a man's quality of life can be substantial. Although medical interventions are of paramount importance in the management of prostatitis, nutrition is frequently disregarded despite its potential to enhance overall health and alleviate symptoms. A comprehensive understanding of the relationship between nutrition and the management of prostatitis is critical for promoting prostate health.

Alternatives To The Prostatitis Lifestyle

Lifestyle modifications can play a crucial role in the management of prostatitis symptoms and the promotion of prostate health as a whole. Key lifestyle modifications to contemplate include the following:

1. Maintaining proper hydration is essential for the health of the prostate. Water aids in the elimination of impurities and supports optimal urinary function,

thereby decreasing the likelihood of complications linked to prostatitis.

2. Anti-inflammatory Dietary Intake: Implementing an anti-inflammatory diet may provide some relief from the symptoms associated with prostatitis. Concentrate on consuming whole cereals, fruits, vegetables, lean proteins, and vegetables. Incorporate omega-3 fatty acid-rich foods, such as fatty salmon, flaxseeds, and hazelnuts, into your diet due to their anti-inflammatory properties.

3. Pelvic floor exercises, such as Kegels, have the potential to enhance blood circulation to the prostate and mitigate the symptoms associated with prostatitis by strengthening the muscles of the pelvic floor.

4. Consistent physical activity can aid in the maintenance of a healthy body weight and the mitigation of inflammation.

Strive to complete a minimum of 150 minutes of exercise per week at a moderate intensity, including leisurely walking, swimming, and cycling.

5. Stress Management: Prostatitis symptoms may be worsened by chronic stress. Daily incorporation of stress-relieving activities such as yoga, meditation, and deep breathing exercises.

6. Limiting Caffeine and Alcohol Consumption Caffeine and alcohol can irritate the prostate and exacerbate symptoms. Particularly in the evening, restricting their intake could potentially aid in the management of prostatitis.

7. In addition to exacerbating symptoms, obesity is associated with an elevated risk of developing prostatitis and should be avoided. Prostate health is dependent upon achieving and maintaining a healthy weight through a balanced diet and regular exercise.

Prostatitis And The Management Of Weight

Effective weight management is an essential component of prostatitis treatment. An increased risk of developing prostatitis is associated with obesity, which can also exacerbate symptoms in those who have already been diagnosed. Weight management can have the following beneficial effects on prostatitis:

1. Inflammation Reduction: Prostatitis symptoms may be exacerbated by chronic inflammation, which is associated with obesity. The maintenance of a healthy body weight has the potential to decrease systemic inflammation, thereby enhancing the health of the prostate.

2. The regulation of hormones: An example of a hormone that can be disrupted by obesity is testosterone, a hormone that influences prostate health. In addition to promoting hormonal stability, weight management techniques such as consistent

exercise and a well-balanced diet can be of assistance.

3. Enhanced Blood Flow: An unhealthy blood circulation is a complication of obesity, which can have detrimental effects on the health of the prostate.

A healthy weight maintained through consistent exercise facilitates optimal blood circulation to the prostate, thereby contributing to the management of symptoms.

4. Reduced Urinary Symptoms: Urinary complications, which are prevalent in cases of prostatitis, may be exacerbated by obesity. Potential benefits of weight loss include reduced bladder pressure and enhanced urinary function.

5. Weight management has the potential to augment the efficacy of medical interventions employed in the treatment of prostatitis. Those who maintain a healthy weight may exhibit enhanced responsiveness to medications and achieve more favorable outcomes.

CHAPTER FOUR

Recipes For Meals Suitable For Prostatitis

Promoting prostate health through the consumption of nutrient-dense foods is the essence of a prostatitis-friendly diet. The following recipes are both delectable and nutritious:

1. Quinoa and Salmon Bowl:

• Salmon that has been grilled (high in omega-3 fatty acids)

Quinoa, which is rich in fiber and protein,

• Carrots, broccoli, and bell peppers that have been roasted

• Dressing with olive oil and lemon (anti-inflammatory)

2. Curry with Turmeric Chicken Stir-Fry:

• Chicken breast segment portions

• Anti-inflammatory turmeric

• A combination of bell peppers, broccoli, and snap peas

• Brown rice (abundant in fiber)

3. Chili Vegetate:

• Kidney legumes (high in protein and fiber)

• Bell peppers, shallots, and tomatoes

• Cumin and chili powder (anti-inflammatory)

• Quinoa or rice made with whole grains

4. YOGURT Parfait In Greece:

• Greek yogurt (protein-rich)

• Berries (antioxidant-rich)

• Walnuts or almonds (an excellent source of omega-3 fatty acids)

A thin layer of honey

Illustrative Meal Plans

It is essential to develop diet plans that are both balanced and suitable for individuals with prostatitis to ensure optimal nutrition. The following are examples of menu plans:

(1) Meal Plan:

• Oatmeal topped with berries and a pinch of chia seeds for breakfast.

• Greek yogurt with hazelnuts as a snack.

• A salad consisting of grilled chicken, mixed greens, and a lemon-turmeric vinaigrette for lunch.

Snack: apple slices spread with peanut butter.

• Baked salmon served with quinoa and roasted vegetables for supper.

Two-Meal Plan:

• Whole-grain crostini topped with poached eggs and avocado for breakfast.

Cottage cheese with pineapple pieces serves as a snack.

• Lentil soup accompanied by whole-grain wafers for lunch.

• Snack: hummus spread on carrot spears.

• Tofu stir-fried with brown rice, broccoli, and bell peppers for supper.

In summary, the implementation of a comprehensive strategy for managing prostatitis, encompassing modifications to one's lifestyle, diligent weight control, and adherence to a diet that is suitable for the condition, can substantially enhance general health and wellness.

Through deliberate decision-making regarding diet and daily routines, individuals can promote prostate health and augment the efficacy of medical interventions.

It is imperative to consistently seek personalized guidance from healthcare professionals to address individual health requirements.

Optimal Prostate Health Through Nourishing

Prostatitis, an inflammatory condition affecting the prostate organ, is a prevalent health concern among males worldwide. Although medical intervention is of the utmost importance, the integration of a balanced and targeted nutritional regimen can make a substantial contribution to symptom management and the promotion of general prostate health. This article will explore three fundamental components of the nutrition of individuals with prostatitis: natural and herbal remedies, professional consultation and guidance, and frequently asked questions (FAQs).

Leveraging The Potential Of Natural And Herbal Remedies To Promote Prostate Health

1. Saw Palmetto: Regarding prostatitis, saw palmetto (Serenoa repens) is a widely recognized herbal remedy. This natural supplement, derived from the berries of the saw palmetto plant, has been the subject of scientific investigation due to its purported

ability to mitigate symptoms including inflammation and urinary tract issues. It is hypothesized to function by impeding the transformation of testosterone into dihydrotestosterone (DHT), a hormone that is linked to the enlargement of the prostate. Nevertheless, before integrating saw palmetto into your regimen, it is imperative that you seek the advice of a healthcare professional, particularly if you are concurrently using other medications.

2. Quercetin, a flavonoid discovered in an assortment of fruits and vegetables, is notable for its anti-inflammatory and antioxidant characteristics. Research indicates that it might be effective in mitigating prostate inflammation and alleviating symptoms related to prostatitis. Apples, onions, citrus fruits, verdant greens, and other foods are quercetin-rich. Although augmenting one's dietary consumption is advantageous, exercising prudence when considering quercetin supplements is advised;

consulting a healthcare professional is likewise advised.

3. Zinc is a vital mineral that is indispensable for the maintenance of prostate health. It is present in the prostate organ in elevated concentrations and is implicated in a multitude of physiological processes. Zinc supplementation may mitigate the symptoms of prostatitis, according to some studies; however, excessive consumption may result in adverse effects. Including zinc-rich foods in a well-balanced diet, such as whole grains, legumes, and pumpkin seeds, can be a safer and more sustainable method to promote prostate health.

4. Lycopene, an exceptionally potent antioxidant, is copiously present in tomatoes. Lycopene may have a protective effect against prostate inflammation and cancer, according to scientific research. Incorporating lycopene into one's diet can be accomplished in a delectable and nutritious manner by consuming fresh or cooked tomatoes.

Nonetheless, for nutritional benefits, it is vital to maintain a varied diet and not rely solely on one food item.

5. Omega-3 fatty acids, which are prevalent in fatty fish such as mackerel, salmon, and flaxseeds, demonstrate anti-inflammatory characteristics. Consuming these particular foods could potentially aid in the mitigation of inflammation that is commonly linked to prostatitis. Moderation is essential, as overconsumption of omega-3 supplements may result in negative side effects. Dietary balance continues to be vital for overall health.

CHAPTER FIVE

Expert Opinion And Consultation: Exploring The Dietary Terrain

1. Tailored Dietary Strategies: Prostatitis is a multifactorial ailment that is influenced by an array of elements. For individualized dietary recommendations, it is advisable to consult with a registered dietitian or nutritionist, among other professionals. In developing an individualized nutrition plan, these professionals may take into account your specific prostatitis symptoms, general health, and dietary preferences.

2. Observation of Trigger Foods: Certain foods may aggravate the symptoms of prostatitis in some individuals. Although a universal solution does not exist, common triggers consist of caffeinated beverages, piquant foods, and alcohol. By documenting symptom changes and keeping a food journal, it is possible to identify particular foods that may require restriction or avoidance.

Without professional guidance, however, eliminating complete food categories may result in nutritional deficiencies.

3. Prostate Health and Adequate Hydration: Maintaining adequate hydration is vital for overall health, which includes prostate health. Water supports normal physiological functions and aids in the elimination of contaminants. Ensuring sufficient hydration can additionally mitigate urinary symptoms that are linked to prostatitis. However, nocturia (nocturnal urination frequency) can be exacerbated by excessive fluid consumption, particularly in the hours leading up to slumber; therefore, a balanced approach is advised.

4. Supplement Safety: Although natural and herbal supplements may offer potential benefits, it is crucial to exercise caution when utilizing them. Without professional guidance, self-prescribing large doses of supplements or combining multiple supplements may result in adverse effects or drug interactions.

Qualified nutritionists and healthcare professionals can assist in determining appropriate dosages and ensuring the safety of supplements.

FAQs Regarding Prostatitis Nutrition: Responses To Frequent Questions

1. Can prostatitis be cured by diet alone? Although a balanced diet is essential for overall health, it is improbable that it will be sufficient to cure prostatitis. Prostatitis is a complex medical condition that frequently necessitates a holistic strategy encompassing dietary support, lifestyle adjustments, and medical intervention.

2. How Long Do Dietary Modifications Take to Produce Results? The rate of progress differs among individuals. While certain individuals may observe a delayed onset of symptom relief following the adoption of dietary modifications, others may demand a longer period. It is essential to adhere to a balanced diet consistently and to seek regular assessments from healthcare professionals.

3. Are nutritional supplements required for prostatitis? Although supplementation can be advantageous, it is not always required. A varied and comprehensive dietary regimen has the potential to supply vital nutrients that are crucial for prostate health. Supplements ought to be evaluated in the presence of a professional, and exclusive reliance on them is not advised.

4. Are Certain Foods Prostatitis Patients Should AVOID? Although the list of trigger foods can differ among individuals, general advice suggests limiting alcohol, caffeine, fiery foods, and alcohol.

In most cases, however, complete avoidance of entire dietary categories is not mandatory. Particular dietary restrictions must be identified through a specialized procedure supervised by a medical professional.

5. Can Exercise and Body Weight Influence Prostatitis Symptoms? Consistently engaging in physical activity and maintaining a healthy weight

are essential components of overall health, including prostate health. Exercising may reduce the risk of developing prostatitis and mitigate its symptoms, according to studies. A healthful lifestyle in conjunction with dietary modifications can contribute to optimal health.

In summary, the management of prostatitis nutrition necessitates a deliberate integration of natural and herbal remedies, expert advice, and the provision of frequently asked questions (FAQs). By incorporating these components into a comprehensive strategy, one can promote prostate health, mitigate symptoms, and enhance overall well-being.

Nevertheless, it is imperative to customize these approaches for each individual and consult a healthcare professional to guarantee a secure and efficacious trajectory in the management of prostatitis.

Conclusion

In summary, nutrition is an essential factor in the prevention and management of prostatitis, a prevalent and frequently incapacitating ailment that impacts the prostate. By incorporating a nutritious diet that is abundant in fruits, vegetables, and whole cereals, one can enhance the overall health of the prostate. Potentially reducing the risk of prostatitis, antioxidants present in fruits and vegetables, such as lycopene in tomatoes, may exert protective effects on the prostate.

It is critical to maintain a healthy weight by adhering to a balanced diet and engaging in consistent physical activity, as obesity has been associated with an elevated likelihood of developing prostatitis.

Moreover, maintaining adequate hydration supports urinary function and aids in the elimination of impurities from the body, which may reduce prostate inflammation.

It is advisable for individuals diagnosed with prostatitis to restrict their consumption of irritants, including caffeine, alcohol, and piquant foods, as these substances have the potential to worsen symptoms. The prospective anti-inflammatory properties of omega-3 fatty acids, which are present in flaxseeds and fish, could facilitate alleviation for certain individuals afflicted with prostatitis.

It is of the utmost importance that individuals afflicted with prostatitis symptoms seek the advice of a healthcare professional to obtain a comprehensive management strategy that incorporates nutritional guidance. Although nutrition may not possess curative properties, it can serve as a supplementary factor in mitigating symptoms and fostering prostate well-being.

In general, individuals with prostatitis may benefit from a healthier lifestyle and a potential enhancement in quality of life through the adoption of a balanced and conscientious approach to nutrition.

THE END

www.ingramcontent.com/pod-product-compliance
Lightning Source LLC
Chambersburg PA
CBHW050703250726
48662CB00002B/817